Pharmacology Laboratory Manual

Pharmacy & Clinical Pharmacology

Second Edition

VOLUME 2

K.C. Singhal

M.D., Ph.D. (Med.), F.I.A.N., F.I.A.M.S.

Professor

Department of Pharmacology

J.N. Medical College, A.M.U.,

Aligarh - 202 002

CBSPD

CBS Publishers & Distributors Pvt Ltd

New Delhi • Bengaluru • Chennai • Kochi • Kolkata • Lucknow • Mumbai

Gujarat • Hyderabad • Jharkhand • Nagpur • Patna • Pune • Uttarakhand

Disclaimer

Science and technology are constantly changing fields. New research and experience broaden the scope of information and knowledge. The author have tried their best in giving information available to them while preparing the material for this book. Although, all efforts have been made to ensure optimum accuracy of the material, yet it is quite possible some errors might have been left uncorrected. The publisher, the printer and the author will not be held responsible for any inadvertent errors, omissions or inaccuracies.

Pharmacology Laboratory Manual

Volume 2

Second Edition

ISBN: 978-81-239-0553-2

Second Edition: 1997

Reprint: 1999, 2002, 2003, 2004, 2005, 2006, 2007, 2010, 2013, 2017, 2018, 2019, 2020, 2024, **2026**

First Edition: 1991

Reprint: 1993, 1995

Published by **Satish Kumar Jain** and produced by **Varun Jain** for

CBS Publishers & Distributors Pvt Ltd

4819/XI Prahlad Street, 24 Ansari Road, Daryaganj, New Delhi 110 002, India.
Ph: 011-23266838, 23289259 Website: www.cbspd.com
e-mail: delhi@cbspd.com

Corporate Office: 204 FIE, Industrial Area, Patparganj, Delhi 110 092
Ph: 011-4934 4934 Fax: 011-4934 4935
e-mail: publishing@cbspd.com; publicity@cbspd.com

Branches

- **Bengaluru:** Seema House 2975, 17th Cross, KR Road, Banasankari 2nd Stage, Bengaluru 560 070, Karnataka, India
  Ph: +91-80-26771678/79 Fax: +91-80-26771680 e-mail: bangalore@cbspd.com
- **Chennai:** 18/8B, Subbaraya Street, Shenoy Nagar, Chennai 600 030, Tamil Nadu, India
  Ph: +91-044-42032115, 044-26681266 e-mail: chennai@cbspd.com
- **Kochi:** 42/1325, 1326, Power House Road, Opp KSEB, Power House, Ernakulum Kochi 682 018, Kerala, India
  Ph: +91-484-4059061-65,67 Fax: +91-484-4059065 e-mail: kochi@cbspd.com
- **Kolkata:** 147, Hind Ceramics Compound, 1st Floor, Nilgunj Road, Belghoria, Kolkata-700056, West Bengal, India
  Ph: +033-25633055, 033-25633056 e-mail: kolkata@cbspd.com
- **Lucknow:** Basement, Khushnuma Complex, 7 Meerabai Marg (Behind Jawahar Bhawan), Lucknow-226001, UP, India
  Ph: +0522-4000032 e-mail: tiwari.lucknow@cbspd.com
- **Mumbai:** PWD Shed, Gala no 25/26, Ramchandra Bhatt Marg, Next to JJ Hospital Gate no. 2, Opp. Union Bank of India, Noorbaug, Mumbai-400009, Maharashtra, India
  Ph: 022-66661880/89 e-mail: mumbai@cbspd.com

Representatives

- Gujarat 0-9879558667
- Hyderabad 0-9885175004
- Jharkhand 0-9811541605
- Nagpur 0-8692091830
- Patna 0-9334159340
- Pune 0-9664372571
- Uttarakhand 0-9716462459

Printed at Rashtriya Printer, Delhi, India

PREFACE

There has been a rethinking during the past decade that the syllabus and the method of teaching of pharmacology are at variance with bed side medical practice. It is therefore not surprising that teachers in this discipline are blamed of bothring little to identify the needs of the undergraduate medical student or of not making any serious attempt to revitalize the concept of relevant teaching/ training. Such rethinking has prompted the author to reframe the list of practicals/ demonstrations with the concurrence of teachers from several medical colleges in the country.

The purpose of laboratory techniques in Pharmacology is to develop a scientific foundation for the use of drugs in the prevention, diagnosis and treatment of disease. In these manuals, an attempt has been made to acquaint the undergraduate medical student with the experimental approach to the science of Pharmacology. On the basis of recommendation of Indian Pharmacological Society expert committee for revision of undergraduate curriculum in pharmacology, some conventional practicals which had lost relevance have been deleted and new ones like ADR monitoring, essential drug list, clinical pharmacology experiments, rationale use of drugs, dissolution, disintegration and hardness of tablets have been added.

An attempt is made to give the student an insight into the action of the more important therapeutic agents and to enable him, from the experiments outlined, to grasp the clinical applications of Pharmacology.

The author gratefully acknowledges the help, cooperation and constructive criticism of all the teachers, colleagues and friends in Pharmacology Departments from many medical colleges. Special thanks are due to Dr. Anil Kumar, Dr. Hemant K. Garg and my wife Prof. (Mrs.) Usha Singhal for useful suggestions. Thanks are due to Mr. Subhash Varshney for managing press materials.

1997
Aligarh - 202 002
India

K.C. Singhal

Name...

Session..

Class Roll No..

Batch ....

Name of the Department & Institution ....

....

....

CERTIFICATE

This is to certify that Mr./Ms..

....has

completed course of practicals in Pharmacy & Clinical Pharmacology/ Experimental Pharmacology satisfactorily.

Date .... **Teacher Incharge**

CONTENTS

PRESCRIPTION ORDER WRITING

The prescription order is an important therapeutic transaction between physician and patient. It brings into focus the diagnostic acumen and therapeutic proficiency of the physician with instructions for palliation or restoration the patient's health. The most carefully conceived prescription order may become therepeutically useless, however, unless it communicates clearly with the pharmacist and adequately instructs the patient on how to take the prescribed medication

The practice of writing complex prescription orders containing many active ingradients, adjuvants, correctives and vehicles is no longer used. Single drugs and mixture of drugs compounded by pharmaceutical companies are usually prescribed. Prescribing fixed dose combinations although may be desirable in some situations because of ease but simplicity has its drawbacks. It does not allow the physician to adjust the dose of each ingredient.

Prescription should be written legibly in ink or type written, dated and signed by the prescriber, and the full name and address of the individual patient added. The age of the patient should preferably be stated, and is legal requirement in the case of prescription - only medicinces for children. In general practice the following should be noted.

Choice of Drug Name

The drugs can be prescribed by their non proprietary (generic) names or by the manufacturer's proprietary (brand) names. In writing prescription it is best to use the nonproprietary name followed by the name of manufacturer in parentheses if a specific manufacturer's product has distinct advanges.

Choice of System for Weights and Measures.

Prescription order should always be written in metric system. Sometimes the drugs, usually syrups, are prescribed in terms of household measures like teaspoon or tablespoonful. Since the size of houshold spoons also varies considerably the pharmacopea specifies that teaspoon may be regarded as containing 5 ml. A tablespoon is said to contain 15ml.

1. (a) For solids, quantities of 1 gram or more should be written as 1 g etc.

   (b) Quantities less than 1 gram should be written in milligrams, e.g. 500 mg, not 0.5 g.

   Quantities less than 1 mg should be written in micrograms e.g. 100 micrograms, not 0.1 mg.

2. When decimals are unavoidable a zero should be written in front of the decimal point where there is no other figure, e.g. 0.5 ml, not .5 ml.

3. Micrograms and nanograms should not be abbreviated. Similarly units should not be abbreviated.

4. The term mililitre (ml) is used in medicine and pharmacy, and cubic centimetre c.c. or cm^3 should not be used.

5. Dose and dose frequency should be stated

Construction of Prescription Order

Prescription always follows a definite pattern. This remains the same whether the prescription is for single drug, Drug combination or mutiple drugs. The elements of prescription are shown in the following example.

May 5, 1997

1.

2. ABC, Age 26 Yr.
16/39 Begum Bridge
Meerut

3. R

4. Digoxin Tablet
(Burroughs Welcome Co.) 0.25 mg

5. Dispense 100 tablets

6. Label : Take 1 tablet at 9.00 A.M. each morning
Digoxin, 0.25 mg. 100 tablets.

7. Do not refill.

8.

A.K.S.,M.D.

1. Date : The date when the prescription order is written is important
2. Name, Address and Age of the Patient
3. The symbol R (not Rx) is an abbreviation for recipe, the latin for "take thou"
4. Drug, strength, and inert additives.

The body of the prescription order contains the name and strength (dose) of the drug. Abbreviations should be avoided lest they may result in prescribing error. In formulations with more than one ingradient the principal drug (which gives the prescription its chief action) is written first followed by the vehicle, the solvent for a solution or the bulking agent for a capsule, goes last.

5. Directions to the Pharmacist.

For Such drug the order consits of "Dispense 10 tablets," "Dispense 200 ml." and so forth.

For two or more drugs the order is usually a short sentence such as "Make a solution", or "Mix and place into 10 Capsules" or a word such as "Mix".

6. Directions to the patient

Should always be written in English or in a language the patient understands. Expressions like "take as directed", are never satisfactory and should be avoided. The direction to the patient contain instructions as to the amount of drug to be taken, the time and frequency of the dose, and other factors such as dilution and route of administration. If a device is involved in the administration of the medication the physician and/or pharmacist should demostrate how it is used. If the drug is to be used externally only, or to be shaken well before using, or if it is a poison, such facts are included.

If the drug is to be taken at a specific time of day or taken three or four times a day, the exact time or times should be specified on the lable. To avoid error the directions for a preparation for internal use should start with a word ***take***, for an ointment or lotion, the word ***apply***, for suppositories, the word ***insert***, and for drops to be placed in the conjunctival sac, external auditory canal or nostril, the word ***place***.

7. Refill Information

Write "Do Not Refill" when the prescription should not be repeated, which is the care in most of the situations. This is intended to control overuse, and abuse of prescription medicine,

8. Signature : Prescription order should be signed, by the physician at the bottom with professional degree, Address and Registration number.

DOSES CALCULATION

Drug doses are usually stated in mg/kg body weight and may be calculated as follows.

mg/kg x body weight (kg) = individual's dose

Drug doses may also be stated in units; e.g. vitamin A and D, some antibiotics and hormones. This means that a certain quantity of biological activity of that drug is called 1 unit. The units are calculated based on Pharmacological assay procedures and reference standards.

Various rules for calculating the doses for infant and children have been devised. Most of them give only approximate dosages because they erroneously assume that child is a small adult. Children are sometimes more susceptible to drugs and doses based on pharmacokinetic studies or clinical experiences mentioned in the text books of Pharmacology or Paediatrics should instead be followed.

Rules for the Infants and Children's Doses (approximate only)

1. **Young's Rule** (for children 2 years and older)

$$\frac{\text{Age (yr)}}{\text{Age (yr)} + 12} \times \text{adult dose}$$

2. **Clark's Rule**

$$\frac{\text{Weight (lb)}}{150} \times \text{adult dose}$$

3. **Fried's Rule** (for infants and children upto 2 years old)

$$\frac{\text{Age (months)}}{150} \times \text{adult dose}$$

4. **The square Meter Surface Area Method**

This may be a more realisitic way of relating dosages

$$\frac{\text{Body surface area of child}}{\text{Body surface area of adult}} \times \text{adult dose}$$

The average body surface area for an adult is taken as 1.73 square meters. Given below is a table indicating fraction of adult dose for a child based on surface area of average adult (1.73 M^2).

Weight in Kg	Age (approx)	Surface area M^2	Percentage of adult dose
2		0.15	09
4		0.25	14
6	3 mths	0.33	19
8		0.40	23
10	1 yr	0.46	27
15		0.63	36
20	5 yr	0.83	48
25		0.95	55
30	9 yr	1.08	62
35		1.20	69
40	12 yr	1.30	75
70	adult	1.76	100

Surface area is roughly determined from the body weight and age and dose is calculated by the following relation.

$$\text{Dose} = \text{Adult dose} \ \frac{\text{Surface area } (M^2) \times 60}{100}$$

OR

$$\text{Dose} = \text{Adult dose} \ \frac{\text{Surface area of child } (M^2)}{1.76}$$

EXPERIMENT No. 1

Absorption, is the entry of drug molecules into the blood via the mucous membranes of the alimentary or respiratory tract or from the site of injection. The speed and total amount of drug absorbed is dependent upon many factors of which the route of absorption is the most important. Advantage is taken of these factors to modify the fate of drug according to patient's requirement. The rate of absorption determines to a large extent the speed of onset and the magnitude and duration of action. The rate of administration is also important for determining the rate of absorption. Intravenous administration eliminates factors concerned with absorption and the effect occurs almost instantaneously.

Objective :

To demonstrate that the rate of drug absorption differs with the route of administration.

Procedure :

1. Select six rats weighing 120 to 150 g.
2. Administer sodium pentobarbitone 30 mg/kg to five rats by different routes as shown in table below. The sixth rat is administered equal volume of saline and serves as control.
3. At intervals gently placethe rat on its back. Inability of the rat to resume upright posture indicates loss of righting reflex.
4. Note the time of drug administration, loss of righting reflex and the time when the reflex is regained.

Effect of route of administration on rate of absorption of sodium pentobarbitone

Rat No.	Route	Loss of righting reflex	
		Time of onset	Time of recovery
1.	Oral		
2.	Subcutaneous		
3.	Intramuscular		
4.	Intraperitoneal		
5.	Intravenous		
6. Control	Normal saline		

Inference :

Absorption is fatest by .... route.
Absorption is slowest by .... route.
Duration of action is longest by .... route and slowest by .... route.

EXPERIMENT No. 2

Excretion is defined as removal of the original drug molecule or its metabolites from the body.A drug can be excreted unaltered by several routes such as saliva, sweat, bile, urine and bowels. A drug may be uniformly distributed in various body fluids or concentrated in a particular tissue for which it has high affinity e.g. ampicillin for gall bladder, iodides for thyroid, digoxin for myocardium, penicillin for kidneys. Kidney diisease can prolong duration of action of a drug by retarding excretion. There is many fold variation in the rate of excretion of drugs. The time taken for original drug concentration to be halved is called 'Half Life'. Some drugs like lignocaine, sodium nitroprusside have short half lives while others like digoxin have long half lives.

Objective :

To demonstrate the variation in rate of excretion of drugs.

Procedure :

1. Students who are ill or allergic to drug should not participate.
2. Preserve a control specimen of saliva and urine.
3. Each student will ingest one of the following drugs :
   (a) Potassium iodide 0.3 g
   (b) Sulphadiazine 0.5 g with 1 g sodium bicarbonate
   (c) Mixture containing 1 g sodium salicylate and 0.6 g sodium bicarbonate, one dose.
4. Drink 250 ml water after drug ingestion.
5. Collect saliva and urine samples every half an hour.
6. The following tests are carried out :

   (a) Iodides - To a sample of urine or saliva add a small amount of sodium nitrate solution and dilute sulphuric acid. A yellow brown colour changing to blue on addition of starch solution constitutes a positive test for iodides.

   (b) Salicylates - (i) To 3 ml urine add 1% ferric chloride solution. The phenol reaction is hindered by acids. Try this with 0.1% solution of sodium salicylate.

   (ii) To 3 ml urine add a drop of dilute sodium hydroxide solution, heat gently; neutralize carefully to litmus with hydrochloric acid, cool and test as in (i). This is especially useful for estors of salicylic acid.

(c) Sulphonamides - immerse in urine a test paper impregnated with diethylaminobenzaldehyde. a colour reaction will appear on the paper. Determine the percentage by matching this with standard paper. Repeat the test with saliva sample.

Record your observations as below :

Excretion of Drugs

Time	Salicylates in urine		Sulphonamide		Iodide	
	Free	Ester	Urine	Saliva	Urine	Saliva
Control						
After 30 mins.						
After 60 mins.						
After 90 mins.						
After 120 mins.						

- negative test + to ++++ positive response.

compare result with other students.

DOSE CALCULATION IN RENAL DISEASES

Estimation of GFR is the most critical evaluation required for ascertaining renal function. The methods used include the following.

A. Insulin clearance test.

B. Creatinine clearance test - Creatinine is estimated in 24 hr. urine sample. The creatinine in urine should approximate creatinine production, low clearance indicate renal in sufficiency. The normal value for an adult 75 in steady state is 20 mg/kg/day.

C. Serum creatinine - It is by far the most frequently used indicator of glomerular function. A number of formulas and normograms have been derived for both children and adults by which to predict the GFR, using the serum creatinine concentration, age and body weight in adults.

For males

$$\text{GFR (ml/min)} = \frac{[140\text{-Age-yr})] \times [\text{body wt. in kg}]}{72 \times \text{serum creatinine mg/dl}}$$

For women the calculated value is multiplied by 0.85.

Dosage Calculation :

For drugs with substantial renal elimination, dosage calculation should be individualized when renal failure is present. This estimate is often made by grouping the degree of renal dysfunction with mild, moderate and severe categories in the following manner.

Mild - GFR = > 50 ml/min

Moderate - GFR = 10-50 ml/min

Severe - GFR < 10 ml/min

PRINCIPLES OF DOSAGE MODIFICATION

1. A very precise modification of dosage regimen is clearly not important for drugs that have minor or insignificant adverse effects or are cleared rapidly by non renal routes e.g. Penicillin G, Doxycycline.
2. No mathematical formula will prevent ADRs when the drug is very toxic, especially when therapeutic index is small.
3. Ideally modification of dosage regimen should produce serum concentration.

DRUGS TO BE AVOIDED IN RENAL IMPAIRMENT

Acetazolamide

Acetohexamide

Amantadine

Nonsteroidal antiinflammatory drugs including Aspirin

Bacampicillin

Bethanidine

Carbenoxolone

Cephalothin

Chloramphenicol

Choloroquine

Chlorthazide

Chlorpropamide

Cisplatin

Clofibrate

Codein

Colchicin

Cycloserin

Debrisoquine

Dextromethorphan

Dextropropoxyphene

Ergotamine

Ethacrynic Acid

Ethambutol

Gallamine

Glibenclamide

Gold salts

Lithium

Magnesium salts

Metformin

Methocarbamol

Metoclopramide

Morphine

Nalidixic Acid

Neomycin

Nitrofurantoin

Penicillamine

Pethidine

Pivampicillin

Primidone

Probenecid

Sodium nitroprusside

Sulindac

Sulfadiazine

Sulphinpyrazone

Talampicillin

Tetracyclines (except Doxycyclin or Minocyclin)

Thiazide diurectics

MIXTURES

Mixtures are aqueous liquid preparations which contain suspended, insoluble, solid substances and are intended for oral administration. The insoluble substances do not make the mixture very viscous and the particles may be held in suspension by the use of suitable suspending or thickening agents. Newer agents like carboxy methylcellulose are now being used for the purpose.

CARMINATIVE MIXTURE

A carminative is a volatile oil (in a drug, liquor or candy) which is able to relieve the feeling of discomfort and distension after food by aiding in the eructation or movement of gases from the stomach. They may also induce relaxation of cardiac sphincters.

For A B C

Sodium bicarbonate	1.3 gm
Tincture cardamom co.	2.0 ml
Spirit ammonia aromaticus	1.0 ml
Spirit chloroform	1.0 ml
Add water to	30.0 ml

Make a mixture send such three doses

One dose three times a day after meals

How do different ingradients of the mixture act as carminative

Sodium Bicarbonate : Serves as basis, acts as carminative and antacid. By interaction with HCl of stomach carbon dioxide is liberated which causes stimulation folowed by contraction of fundus of stomach and gases are expelled by eructation.

$$NaHCO_3 + HCl = NaCl + H_2O + CO_2$$

Tincture cardamom compound : Acts as an adjuvant. Its components including cardamom, caraway and cochineal (wings of female insect Doetylopus) act as carminative antispasmodic and provide flavour to mixture. Cochineal also imparts red colour to mixture.

Spirit ammonia aromaticus : Acts as carminative and antispasmodic.

Spirit chloroform : Acts as antispasmodic.

Contraindication :

- Diseases requiring sodium restriction.
- Pyloric obstruction.
- Peptic ulcer.

[15]

Prescription Writing and Notes

POWDERS

ORAL REHYDRATION POWDER

Diarrhoea may cause metabolic acidosis whereas vomiting may result in metabolic alkalosis hypopotassimia. When the fluid and electrolyte loss is severe intravenous infusion becomes essential.

To compensate the loss of fluid and ions in diarrohea and also in vomiting Oral Rehydration Salt dissolved in boiled and cooled water is administered orally. Addition of glucose facilitate the absorption of sodium from intestine and water causes expansion in plasma volume and corrects dehydration.

Loss of electrolytes in diarrhoeal and normal stool

	Na	K	Cl	HCO_3	Volume
			m mol 1^{-1}		litre/day
Normal stool	20-40	30-60	20	-	0.1
Diarrhoea	30-140	30-70	-	20-80	Variable

Changes in body weight of 0.5-1 kg in 24 hours are usually due to loss or gain of water. The following table relates the degree of dehydration to weight loss.

Assessment of dehydration

Dehydration	Fluid loss % body weight	
	Children	Adult
Mild	5	4
Moderate	10	6
Severe	15	8

ORAL REHYDRATION POWDER (O.R.P.)

Ingredients

Sodium chloride		3.5 gm
Sodium bicarbonate		2.5 gm
Potassium chloride		1.5 gm
Glucose		20.0 gm
	Total	27.5 gm

LOTIONS

Lotions are liquid suspensions or dispersions intended for external application for their local effects on skin or mucous membrane. They may be prepared by triturating the ingredients to a smooth paste and then slowly adding the remaining liquid phase. High speed mixes or homogenizers produce better dispersions and are therefore the tools of choice in the preparations of large quantities of lotion. Lotions are usually applied without friction.

CALAMINE LOTION

Calamine lotion is the classical example of lotion and consists of finely powdered, insoluble solids held in more or less permanent suspension by the presence of suspending agents and/or surface active agents.

Ingredients

Calamine		4.5 gm
Zinc oxide		1.5 gm
Bentonite		0.9 gm
Sodium citrate		0.15 gm
Liquified Phenol		0.15 ml
Glycerine		1.5 ml
Distilled water	to	30.0 ml

Shake well before use

apply lotion topically on the affected part two or three times a day, without friction.

Action of ingredients

Calamine : It is zinc oxide with a small proportion of ferric oxide. Action like zinc oxide.

Zinc oxide : Acts as mild astringent, protective and antiseptic.

Sodium citrate : Increase dispersal ability of bentonite. Prevent darkening of the lotion because of iron content.

Bentonite : absorbs water and acts as suspending agents for calamine nd zinc oxide which are water insoluble.

Liquid phenol : antiseptic

Glycerine : emollient (emollier-to soften), keeps the texture of skin soft and smooth.

Water : solvent for sodium citrate, diluent for liquified phenol and glycerine and vehicle for solution.

POTASSIUM PERMANGANATE SOLUTION

Ingredients

Potassium permanganate		100 mg
Water	to	100 ml

Mix and prepare a lotion

It must be freshly prepared.
One part is to be diluted with 7 parts of water, or as directed.
The diluted solution contains potassium permanganate about 1 in 8000.

Uses :

- gargle or mouth wash
- irrigation of ulcer, wound, bladder
- gastric lavage in poisoning due to oral ingestion of barbiturates, alkaloids like morphine, strychnine and picrotoxin
- disinfection of drinking water of wells.

Pharmacological basis of action

Potassium permanganate is a strong oxidising agent. When it comes in contact with skin and water nascent oxygen is released which oxidises bacterial protoplasm and renders it inactive.

[20]

Prescription Writing and Notes

EMULSION

An emulsion is a two-phase system in which one liquid is dispersed in the form of small globules throughout another liquid. The dispersed liquid is known internal phase, whereas dispersion medium is known as the external or continuous phase. When oil is the dispersed and an aqueous solution is the continuous phase, the system is designated as oil-in-water (O/W) emulsion. Conversely, when water or an aqueous solution is the dispersed phase and oil or oleaginous material is the continuous phase, the system is designated as a water-in-oil (W/O) emulsion.

BENZYL BENZOATE EMULSION

Ingredients

Benzyl benzoate		5.25 gm
Emulsifying wax		0.5 gm
Water	to	25.0 ml

Mix and prepare an emulsion

Uses : used as parasiticidal

1. This emulsion is used for the treatment of scabies. It is applied (below neck) with a brush after entire body has been thorougly scrubbed with soft soap and hot water. A second coat is applied when the first is dry and the lotion is left on the body for 24 hours. At the end of that time the body is again thoroughly bathed and dressed in clean cloths. All members of the family are treated simultaneously. Benzyl benzoate is irritant to the skin; application for children should be diluted with 1 volume of water and 3 volumes for infants.
2. Pediculosis - apply 25% application to affected area for 24 hours, remove by washing; in severe cases repeat 2-3 times.

[22]

Prescription Writing and Notes

LINIMENTS

Liniments are liquid or semisolid preparations intended for use over skin. Many of them an solutions or emulsions. They are intended for external application and should be so labelled. Liniments are applied wiith friction and rubbing of the skin, the oil or soap base providing for ease of application and massage. Liniments should not be applied to skin areas that are bruised or broken.

TURPENTINE LINIMENT (I.P.)

Ingredients

Soft soap		4.5 gm
Camphor		2.5 gm
Turpentine oil		32.5 ml
Water	to	50.0 ml

Mix and prepare a liniment

Action of ingredients :

Rubefacients : acts by counter irritation. Counter irritation is comforting in painful lesions of the muscles, tendons, and joints, and in non-articular reheumatism. Soft soap is used as emulsifying agent and provides the ease of application and massage water acts as vehicle. Camphor and turpentine oil act as counter irritants and rubefacients.

Therapeutic use :

- Abdominal visceral pain
- Muscular or joint pain

[24]

Prescription Writing and Notes

PAINTS

Paints are medicated liquid preparations intended for topical application over skin or mucous membrane. These are used for antiseptic, astringent, cosmetic or analgesic actions.

Throat paints are still being used as adjuvants in allergic or infective conditions of mucosa of oropharynx. Mandl's paint is most commonly applied.

MANDL'S PAINT (N.F.I.)

(Iodine Compound paint)

Ingredients

Iodine		0.31 gm
Potassium iodide		0.62 gm
Water		0.62 ml
Menthol oil		0.10 ml
Alcohol (90%)		0.94 ml
Glycerine	to	25.0 ml

To be applied as throat paint three times a day in between meals.

Uses :

- Acute tonsillitis
- Allergic pharyngitis

Action of the ingredients :

Iodine : is widely used as a germicide, fungicide and antiseptic

Potassium iodide : helps in dissolving iodine in solution

Menthol oil + alcohol : gives a cooling sensation to oropharyngeal mucosa

Glycerine : Acts as a vehicle with demulcent property.

Prescription Writing and Notes

OINTMENTS

There are semisolid preparations for external application and of such consistency that they may readily be applied to the skin by inunction and of such composition that they soften, but not necessarily melt, when applied to the body. They serve as vehicles for topical application of medicinal substances and also function as protective and emollient for the skin. They are also knowns as salves or chrismas. An ointment for use in the eye is known as occulentum.

The vehicle of an ointment is known as ointment base. The base may be a fatty substance or a mixture of fats, waxes and oils. The ointment base usually constitutes the major portion of the pharmaceutical preparation and, therefore, may influence the efficacy of the incorporated medicinal substances.

WHITFIELD'S OINTMENT

(Salicylic acid and benzoic acid ointment)

Ingredients

Salicylic acid		0.75 gm
Benzoic acid		1.5 gm
Vaseline	to	25.0 gm

Mix and prepare an ointment.

Direction for use :

Clean the affected part with soap and water.

Apply ointment locally twice a day.

Uses : It was formerly very widely employed as a keratolytic and fungistatic agent and is still frequently prescribed today. It is used in the treatment of epidermophytosis and ringworm of the scalp.

Stratified squamous epithelial cells of skin are bound together by desmosomes and penetrating tonofibrils, both of which largely consist of keratin. Certain fungi especially dermatophytes, utilize keratin and reside in stratum corneum in those places where the degree of hydration and pH are sufficiently high.

Salicylic acid loosen keratin and facilitates removal of stratum corneum. This process is called as desquamation and these substances are called keratolytics. Salicylic acid is beneficial agent in the local treatment of warts, corns, fungus infection and certain forms of eczematoid dermatitis. Tissue cells swell, soften and ultimately desquamate.

Benzoic acid acts as antifungal.

[28]

Prescription Writing and Notes

DISINTEGRATION TEST

Disintegration is defined as the state in which any residue of the tablet, except fragments of insoluble coating remaining on the screen of the test apparatus consists of a soft mass having no palpably firm, unmoistened core.

Disintegration of the "dosage unit", after ingestion, is necessary for the release, dissolution and consequent absorption of its active constituents. The process may be impaired, and the bioavailability of the drug compromised, by basic errors in formulation or manufacture, e.g. a lack of disintegrants, an excess of lubricants, or over-compression. Improper or prolonged storage may have the same effect, owing for instance to the aging of coating or the hardening of tablets.

In the case of solid dosage forms containing active constitutents that are readily soluble in the intestinal contents, demonstrations of the process of disintegration under standardized conditions in-vitro prove a valuable index of its absorbability in-vivo. One or more substances are usually added to a tablet to facilitate its breakup or disintegration after administration. The active ingredient must be released from the tablet matrix as efficiently as possible to allow for a rapid dissolution. Materials serving as disintgrants have been classified as starches, clays, celluloses algins and gums.

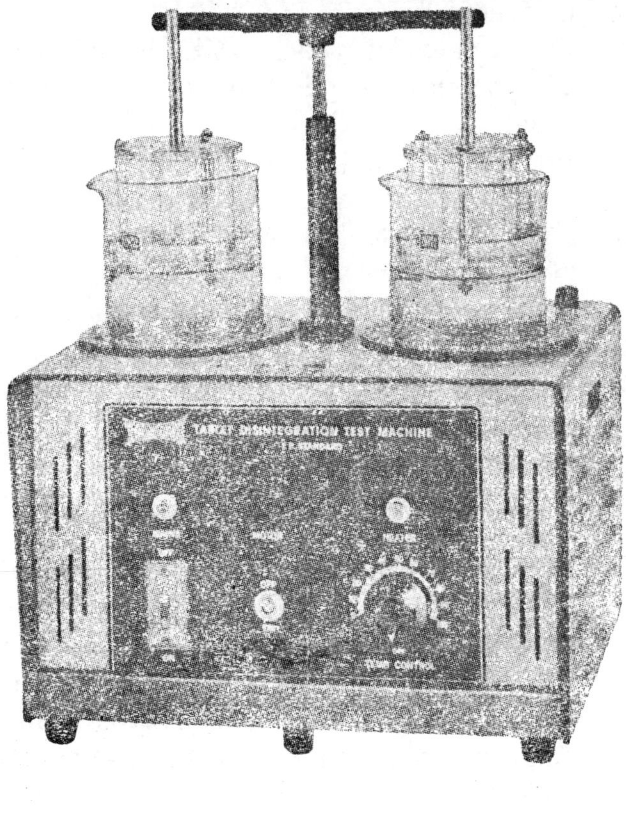

Disintegration test apparatu :

Apparatus is a rigid basket - rack assembly supporting six cylinderical glass tubes.

The tubes are held vertically by two superimposed transparent plastic plates, perforated by six holes having the same diameter as the tubes. The holes are equidistant from the centre of the plate and are equally spaced from one another. Attached to the under side of the lower plate is a piece of woven gauze made from stainless steel wire 635 μm in diameter and having nominal mesh aperture of 2 mm. The upper plate is covered with stainless steel disc perforated with holes to fit over the tubes and hold them between plastic plates. A cylinderical perforated disc made of transparent plastic is provided with each tube.

The assembly is attached to a mechanical device capable of raising and lowering it smoothly at a constant frequency of between 28 and 32 cycles per minute, through a distance of 50 to 60 mm.

The assembly is suspended in the liquid medium. The volume of liquid is such that wire mesh at its highest point is atleast 25 mm below the surface of the liquid and its lowest point is atleast 25 mm above the bottom of the beaker.

Procedure :

(a) Uncoated Tablets :

1. Place one tablet in each of six tubes of the basket, add a disc to each tube, and operate the apparatus using water maintained at 37°C as the immersion liquid.
2. After fifteen minutes, lift the basket from the liquid and observe the tablets.

The tablet pass the test if all the six have disintegrated

3. If one or two tablets fail to disintegrate, repeat the test on 12 additional tablets.

Not less than 16 of the total 18 tablets tested should disintegrate to pass the test.

(b) Enteric coated tablets :

1. Place one tablet in each of the six tubes of the basket. If the tablet has a soluble external coating, immerse the basket in water at room temperature for five minutes.
2. Operate the apparatus, without adding the discs, using 0.1N hydrochloric acid as the immersion liquid maintained at 37°C.
3. At the end of two hours, remove the assembly from the liquid. (No tablet should show signs of either disintegration, apart from fragments of coating, or cracks that would allow the escape of the contents).
4. Add a disc to each tube and operate the apparatus using mixed phosphate buffer pH 6.8 as the immersion liquid maintained at 37°C.
5. At the end of 60 min remove the assembly from the liquid and observe the tablets.

Tablets pass the test if all six have disintegrated

6. If one or two tablets fail to disintegrate, repeat the test on twelve additional tablets. (Not less than 16 of the total 18 tablets tested should disintegrate to pass the test).

(c) Capsules :

The test can also be applied for capsules. Operate the apparatus for 30 mts in case of hard capsules and for sixty minutes in case of soft capsules. The capsules pass the test if no residue remains on the screen of the apparatus or, if a residue remains, it consists of fragments of shell or is a soft mass with no palpable core.

Report Sheet - Disintegration Time of Tablets/Capsules

Proprietary name .... Usual strength ....
Generic name .... Dose ....
Storage instructions .... Type of tablet ....
Clinical use ....
Batch number .... Manufacturer ....
Date of manufacturer.............................. Date of expiry ....

Proprietary name .... Usual strength ....
Generic name .... Dose ....
Storage instructions .... Type of tablet ....
Clinical use ....
Batch number .... Manufacturer ....
Date of manufacturer.............................. Date of expiry ....

Proprietary name .... Usual strength ....
Generic name .... Dose ....
Storage instructions .... Type of tablet ....
Clinical use ....
Batch number .... Manufacturer ....
Date of manufacturer.............................. Date of expiry ....

Disintegration Test :

Disintegration Time for five tablets, disintegrating as per Indian Pharmacopia method is...........................minutes.

Prescription Writing and Notes

DISSOLUTION TEST

The dissolution properties of drugs have been studied and correlated to their absorption. Microcrystalline particles of a drug provide a much greater surface for dissolution, than similar macroparticles. The surface gets more easily wetted by the solvent and the particles therefore dissolved at a faster rate, yielding solution of higher concentration.

Similarly, a correlation between particle size, rate of dissolution, and oral absorption of drugs such as griseofulvin, chloramphenicol, tolbutamide, spironolactone, medroxyprogesterone acetate, sulfisoxazole and aspirin has been described.

The rate of dissolution of an active ingredient can be altered by several factors e.g.

(i) Compaction during tablet manufacture or capsule filling.

(ii) Hydrophobity imparted by tablet lubricants.

(iii) Adsorption of air on the particle surface.

(iv) Surface change on particle.

Dissolution test apparatus :

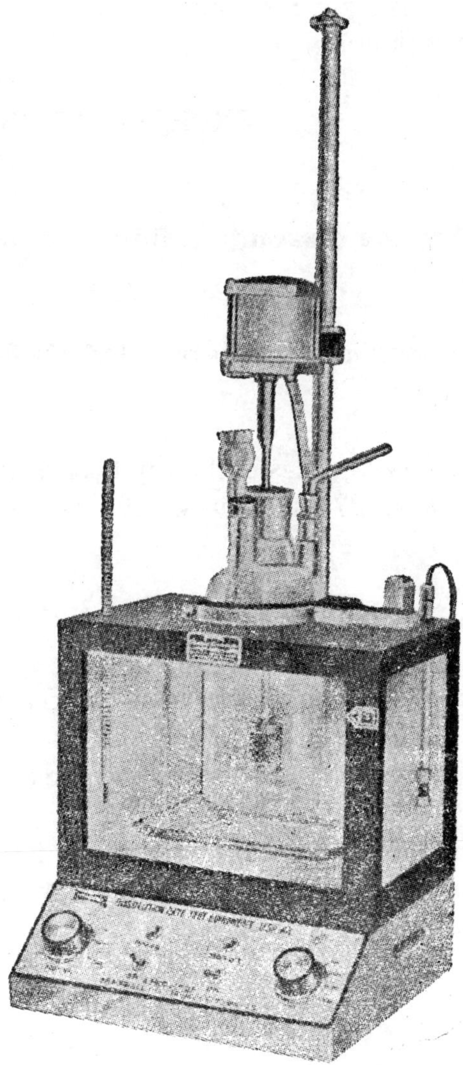

Assembly consists of the folowing :

a) A cyliderical vessel made of glass or any other inert material fitted with a lid which has a number of openings one of which is central.

b) A variable speed motor which causes a basket to rotate in the vessel(25-750 rpm). The shaft passes through the central opening in the lid of the vessel and carries at its lower end a stainless steel disc.

c) A cyliderical stainless steel basket assembly made of woven wire cloth with a nominal aperture of 425 μm. The top of basket is attached to the disc on the driving shaft.

d) The vessel is equipped with a suitable device for the withdrawl of samples of the dissolution medium.

EXPERIMENT NO. 3

Objective :

To determine the dissolution time of a tablet/capsule.

Procedure :

1. Fill the vessel with 1000 ml of water, free from dissolved air and previously warmed at 37°C.

2. Place tablets capsules in the dry basket. Assemble the apparatus. Keep a distance of 23-27 mm between of basket and bottom interior surface of the vessel.

3. Start the motor.

4. Withdraw sample from the vessel at 45 min or specified interval.

5. Determine the amount of active ingredient.

The requirement of the test are met if the amount of active ingredient in solution is not less than 70 percent of the stated amount.

Report Sheet - Dissolution Time of Tablet/Capsule

Proprietary name	....	Usual strength	....
Generic name	....	Dose	....
Storage instructions	....	Type of tablet	....
		Clinical use	....
Batch number	....	Manufacturer	....
Date of manufacturer	....	Date of expiry	....

Time in minutes	Concentration of active ingredient / 100 ml

Report Sheet - Dissolution Time of Tablet/Capsule

Proprietary name	....	Usual strength	....
Generic name	....	Dose	....
Storage instructions	....	Type of tablet	....
		Clinical use	....
Batch number	....	Manufacturer	....
Date of manufacturer	....	Date of expiry	....

Time in minutes	Concentration of active ingredient / 100 ml

Report Sheet - Dissolution Time of Tablet/Capsule

Proprietary name	....	Usual strength	....
Generic name	....	Dose	....
Storage instructions	....	Type of tablet	....
		Clinical use	....
Batch number	....	Manufacturer	....
Date of manufacturer	....	Date of expiry	....

Time in minutes	Concentration of active ingredient / 100 ml

Prescription Writing and Notes

HARDNESS OF A TABLET

The resistance of a tablet to chipping, abrasion or breakage under conditions of storage, transportation and handling before usage depends on its hardness. A commonly used rule of thumb describes a tablet to be of proper hardness if it is firm enough to break with a sharp snap when it is held between the second and third fingers and using the thumb as the fulcrum, yet does not break when it falls on the floor. If the tablet is too hard, it may not disintegrate in the required period of time; if it is too soft, it will not withstand the handling during packaging and transportation.

To quantitate the degree of hardness a tablet hardness tester is used. The instrument measures the force required to break the tablet when the force generated by a coil spring is applied diametrically to the tablet. The force is measured in kilograms and a hardness of 4 kg is considered to be minimum for a satisfactory tablet.

EXPERIMENT NO. 4

Objective :

To determine the hardness of a tablet.

Procedure :

1. Place a tablet in the tester.

2. Screw in the plunger to apply force on the tablet.

3. Read the force required to break the tablet directly from the scale on the outer tube or on the dial depending on the type of instrument used. Scale usually ranges from 0-25 kg/cm^2 with each division marked to 1 kg.

4. The force required to break the tablet is expressed in kilogram/centimeter^2

Report Sheet for Tablets

Generic name	....	Usual strength	....
Proprietary name	....	Dose	....
Name of manufacturer	....	Type of Tablet	....
Batch number	....	Clinical use	....
Date of manufacturer	....	Date of expiry	....

Tablet Hardness Determination

Test Instrument........................

Hardness	Tablet number				
	1	2	3	4	5
Kg/Cm²					

Average Hardness of .... tablet is ....kg/Cm².

Report Sheet for Tablets

Generic name	....	Usual strength	....
Proprietary name	....	Dose	....
Name of manufacturer	....	Type of Tablet	....
Batch number	....	Clinical use	....
Date of manufacturer	....	Date of expiry	....

Tablet Hardness Determination

Test Instrument........................

Hardness	Tablet number				
	1	2	3	4	5
Kg/Cm²					

Average Hardness of .... tablet is ....kg/Cm².

DURABILITY OF THE TABLETS

Another approach to determine the durability of tablets from the time of production to time of use is to evaluate its ability to withstand abrasion in packaging, handling and transportation.

The apparatus consists of transparent acrylic sheet drums (single or double) which rotate at a fixed speed (R.P.M.). The drum is equipped with a plastic blade which carries the tablets along with it up to a predetermined height while the drum is rotating and let them slide off. Thus without any hard impact the tablets rub against each other under the same pressure.

Friability test apparatus :

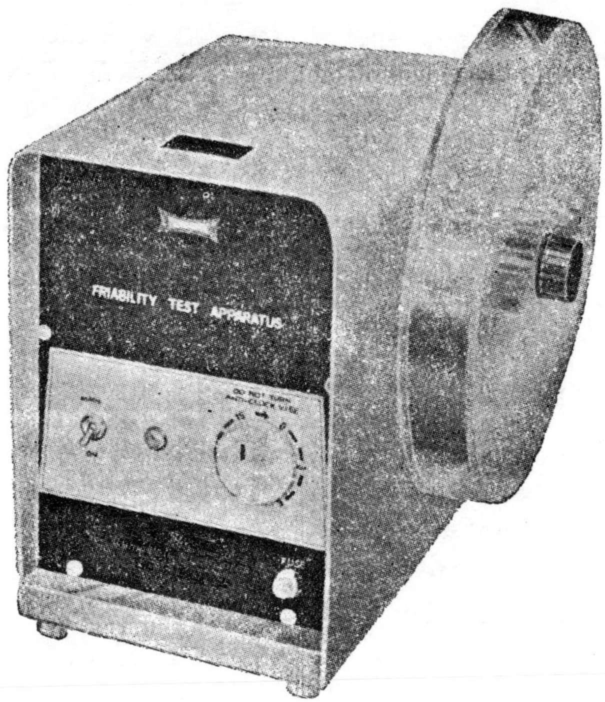

EXPERIMENT NO. 5

Objective : To determine the durability/friability of the tablets.

Procedure :

(a) Weigh a number of tablets.

(b) Place the tablets in the drum of the friability test apparatus.

(c) Switch the apparatus on and run for 15 minute.

(d) Weigh the tablets again

(e) Calculate the percent loss in weight.

- Weight of tablets before (w_1) ....
- Weight of tablets after (w_2) ....
- Loss of weight (w_1-w_2=w_3) ....
- The percent loss in the weight of tablets is $\frac{w_3 \times 100}{w_1}$ ....

(e) Calculate the percent loss in weight.

- Weight of tablets before (w_1) ....
- Weight of tablets after (w_2) ....
- Loss of weight (w_1-w_2=w_3) ....
- The percent loss in the weight of tablets is $\frac{w_3 \times 100}{w_1}$ ....

(e) Calculate the percent loss in weight.

- Weight of tablets before (w_1) ....
- Weight of tablets after (w_2) ....
- Loss of weight (w_1-w_2=w_3) ....
- The percent loss in the weight of tablets is $\frac{w_3 \times 100}{w_1}$ ....

ADVERSE DRUG REACTION MONITORING

The drug that can modify or repress biological processes is invaluable in treatment but if it has this capacity, it is bound also to cause adverse effects. Those who advocate that drug should ensure complete safety demand impossible, as the drug without side effects is probably an ineffective one. The medical profession can not absolve itself from the responsibility. We must confess that there has been a good deal of excessive, irrational, ignorant and irresponsible prescribing.

Adverse Reaction is defined as "A response to a drug which is noxious and unintended, and which occurs at doses normally used in man for the prophylaxis, diagnosis, or therapy of disease,or for the modification of physiological function.

Drugs are marketed prior to compilation of all medically important events. Premarketing studies and clinical trials provide important information on safety and efficacy. However, because of small population size and homogenous population sample, most of the adverse reactions occuring at rates less than one per thousand are usually not detected. Postmarketing surveilleance and ADR monitoring is therefore a necessity.

Although, no common standard for the detailed operational assessment of causality has been agreed upon internationally, However international agreement has recently been reached among participating countries in the WHO drug monitoring scheme on common definitions of the term most often used to describe causality in a semiqualitative way.

WHO Terminology for Causality Assessment.

Causality assessment of suspected Adverse reactions

Certain

A clinical event, including laboratory test abnormality, occuring in a plausible time relationship to drug administration, and which cannot be explained by concurrent disease or other drugs or chemicals. The response to withdrawal of the drug (dechallenge) should be clinically plausible. The event must be definitive pharmacologically or phenomenologically, using a satisfactory rechallenge procedure if necessary.

Probable/Likely

A clinical event, including laboratory test abnormality, with a reasonable time sequence to administration of the drug, unlikely to be attributed to concurrent disease or other drugs or chemicals, and which follows a clinically reasonable response on withdrawal (dechallenge).

Rechallenge information is not required to fulfil this definition.

Possible

A clinical event, including laboratory test abnormality, with reasonable time sequence to administration of the drug, but which could also be explained by concurrent disease or other drugs or chemical. Information on drug withdrawal may be lacking or unclear.

Unlikely

A clinical event, including laboratory test abnormality, with a temporal relationship to drug administration which makes a causal relationship improbable, and in which other drugs, chemicals or underlying disease provide plausible explanations.

Conditional/Unclassified

A clinical event, including laboratory test abnormality, reported as an adverse reaction, about which more data is essential for a proper assessment or the additional data are under examination.

Unassessible/Unclassifiable

A report suggesting a adverse reaction which cannot be judged because information is insufficient or contradictory, and which cannot be supplemented or verified.

Hospitalization due to ADR's

Several studies in Europe, Israel and the US have estimated that 5-10 % of all admittances to acute medical wards are due to ADR's.

Pathogenesis of Adverse Drug Reaction

Types of ADR's

Adverse Reaction can logically and usually clinically be divided into those that arise from normal Pharmacological action of a drug (Type A) and those represent a totally abnormal or novel response (Type B)

Type A ADR's

Are the result of an exaggerated, but otherwise normal Pharmacological action of a drug. These reactions are predictable on the basis or drug's known Pharmacology. They are usually dose dependent and although their incidence and morbidity in the community is often high, their mortality is generally low.

Type B ADR's

Are totally aberrant effects that are unrelated to drug's normal Pharmacology.They are usually unpredicatble and are not observed during conventional Toxicological Sereening Programmes. Although their incidence and morbidity are usually low. their mortality may be high.

Differences between Type A & Type B ADR

	Type A (Augmented response) (Attenuated response)	**Type B** (Bizarre)
Predictable phrmacological	Yes	No
Dose dependent	Yes	No
Incidence & Morbidity	High	Low
Mortality	Low	High
Treatment	Change dose	Stop

Cognizance of the potentials of a drug to cause adverse effects and adequate information about the spectrum and incidence of such effects in given population is essential in balancing the benefits obtained by continued use of the drug against the risks involved. Adverse reactions to drug may be influenced by a large number of socio-economic, genetic, environmental and ethnic factors. In India, these elements might induce a pattern of adverse effects diverse from those seen in other countries and it is unfortunate that we are entirely dependent on ADR data generated abroad. Such adverse reactions reported elswhere may not be strictly and truly applicable in our situation.

Adverse Drug Reaction Monitoring

Name & Address	Age	Sex	Date of Reaction onset	Hospital Record No.

Adverse Reaction	Out Come ☐ A. Recovered without sequelae B. Recovered with sequelae C. Not yet recovered D. Died due to Adverse reaction E. Died drug may be contributory F. Died unrelated to drug G. Unknown

Drugs Trade with Generic Name	Dose	Route	Drug Administration**	
			Began D M Y	Terminated D M Y
1.*				
2.				
3.				
4.				
5.				

* List first the drug suspected to cause reaction

** If exact dates unknown, Record duration

Dechallange ☐

1. Definite improvement
2. No improvement
3. Medication continued
4. Unknown

Rechallange ☐

1. Recurrence of symptoms
2. No recurrence
3. No rechallange performed
4. Unknown

Drug Reaction Relationship ☐

1. Certain
2. Probable
3. Possible
4. Unlikely
5. Unclassified
6. Unclassifiable

Predisposing or contributing conditions.

Adverse Drug Reaction Monitoring

Name & Address	Age	Sex	Date of Reaction onset	Hospital Record No.

Adverse Reaction	Out Come ☐
	A. Recovered without sequelae B. Recovered with sequelae C. Not yet recovered D. Died due to Adverse reaction E. Died drug may be contributory F. Died unrelated to drug G. Unknown

Drugs Trade with Generic Name	Dose	Route	Drug Administration**	
			Began	Terminated
			D M Y	D M Y
1.*				
2.				
3.				
4.				
5.				

* List first the drug suspected to cause reaction

** If exact dates unknown, Record duration

Dechallange ☐

1. Definite improvement
2. No improvement
3. Medication continued
4. Unknown

Rechallange ☐

1. Recurrence of symptoms
2. No recurrence
3. No rechallange performed
4. Unknown

Drug Reaction Relationship ☐

1. Certain
2. Probable
3. Possible
4. Unlikely
5. Unclassified
6. Unclassifiable

Predisposing or contributing conditions.

Adverse Drug Reaction Monitoring

Name & Address	Age	Sex	Date of Reaction onset	Hospital Record No.

Adverse Reaction

Out Come ☐

A. Recovered without sequelae
B. Recovered with sequelae
C. Not yet recovered
D. Died due to Adverse reaction
E. Died drug may be contributory
F. Died unrelated to drug
G. Unknown

Drugs Trade with Generic Name	Dose	Route	Drug Administration**	
			Began D M Y	Terminated D M Y
1.*				
2.				
3.				
4.				
5.				

* List first the drug suspected to cause reaction
** If exact dates unknown, Record duration

Dechallange ☐

1. Definite improvement
2. No improvement
3. Medication continued
4. Unknown

Rechallange ☐

1. Recurrence of symptoms
2. No recurrence
3. No rechallange performed
4. Unknown

Drug Reaction Relationship ☐

1. Certain
2. Probable
3. Possible
4. Unlikely
5. Unclassified
6. Unclassifiable

Predisposing or contributing conditions.

Adverse Drug Reaction Monitoring

Name & Address	Age	Sex	Date of Reaction onset	Hospital Record No.

Adverse Reaction	Out Come ☐
	A. Recovered without sequelae B. Recovered with sequelae C. Not yet recovered D. Died due to Adverse reaction E. Died drug may be contributory F. Died unrelated to drug G. Unknown

Drugs Trade with Generic Name	Dose	Route	Drug Administration**	
			Began D M Y	Terminated D M Y
1.*				
2.				
3.				
4.				
5.				

* List first the drug suspected to cause reaction

** If exact dates unknown, Record duration

Dechallange ☐

1. Definite improvement
2. No improvement
3. Medication continued
4. Unknown

Rechallange ☐

1. Recurrence of symptoms
2. No recurrence
3. No rechallange performed
4. Unknown

Drug Reaction Relationship ☐

1. Certain
2. Probable
3. Possible
4. Unlikely
5. Unclassified
6. Unclassifiable

Predisposing or contributing conditions.

ESSENTIAL DRUGS

Essential drugs are those that satisfy the health care needs of the majority of population; they should therefore be available at all times in adequate amounts and in appropriate dosage forms.

For making optimal use of limited resources, the choice of such drugs depends on many factors such as the pattern of prevalent diseases, the treatment facilities; the training and experience of available personnel; the financial resources, and genetic, demographic and evironmental factors. Only those drugs should be selected for which sound and adequate data on efficacy and safety are available from adequate studies and for which evidence of performance in general use in a variety of medical settings has been obtained.

In the great majority of cases essential drugs should be formulated as single compounds. Fixed ratio combinations products are acceptable only when the dosage of each ingredient meets the requirements of a defined population group and when combination provides a proven advantage over single compounds administered separately in therapeutic effect, safety or compliance.

World Health Organization has provided guidelines for establishing a list of Essential Drugs.

1. Each country should appoint a committee to establish a list of essential drugs.
2. Drug selection should be based on the results of benefit and safety evaluations obtained in controlled clinical trials and/or epidemiological studies.
3. International non proprietary (Generic) names should be used.
4. Selected Pharmaceutical products should meet Quality Control Standards

including stability and when necessary, bioavailability.

5. Cost of treatment must be considered.

6. Competence of prescriber to make correct diagnosis.

7. Influence of local diseases or conditions on pharmacokinetic and pharmacodynamic parameters should be considered in making the selection eg. malnutrition, liver diseases.

8. Highest benefit/risk ratio.

9. When two or more drugs are therapeutically equivalent preference should be given to drug that has been thoroughly investigated, has favourable pharmacokinetic properties, facilities for manufacture and storage exist.

10. Fixed ratio combinations are acceptable only when :

    i. Clinical documentation justifies concomitant use of more than one drug.

    ii. Therapeutic effect is greater than the sum of the effect of each.

    iii. Cost of combination product is less than the sum of individual products.

    iv. Compliance is improved.

    v. Sufficient drug ratio are provided to allow dosage adjustments satisfactory for majority of population.

    vi. The list should be reviewed periodically.

Advantage of the Essential Drug List :

Preparing a rational list of essential/restricted drugs has several advantages: Medical, Economic, Social and Administrative.

Medical Advantages :

1. It is medically, therapeutically and scientifically sound and it ensures rational use of drugs.
2. Limits the use of irrational and hazardous drugs and decreases Drug induced disease.
3. Makes Adverse Drug Reaction Monitoring feasible.

Economic Advantages :

1. Prevents wastage of carse resources on non essentials.
2. Larger production of esssential drugs shall bring down the prices.
3. Curtails aggressive marketing on non essential formulations.

Social Advantages :

1. Responds to real health needs of people.
2. Facilitates dissemination of correct information about drugs.
3. Priorities of drug needs of society can be outlined.

Administrative Advantages :

1. Makes quality control easier.
2. Production, storage and distribution is easy.
3. Price fixation/revision, levying of taxes etc. is facilitated.

Prescription Writing and Notes

ESSENTIAL DRUG LIST

1. Anaesthetics and muscle relaxants & preoperative medication :

1. Anaesthetic ether, liquid, Inhalation
2. Halothane liquid, in 250 ml bottle
3. Lignocaine, inj. 1%, 2% (hydrochloride)
4. Ethlyl chloride, liquid, in 100 ml spray bottles
5. Thiopentone sodium, powder, for inj., 500 mg/ampoule
6. Suxamethonium inj., 50 mg in 2 ml ampoule (chloride)
7. Vancuronium bromide, inj., 10 mg/vial.
8. Pancuronium bromide, inj., 1 mg/ml. 2 mg/ml
9. Atropine inj. 1 mg (sulphate) in 1ml ampoule
10. Diazepam inj. 10 mg (sulphate or hydrochloride) in 1ml ampoule
11. Bupivacaine inj. 2.25%, 0.5% (hydrochloride) in vial
12. Chloral hydrate syrup 200 mg/5 ml

2. Analgesics, antipyretics, non-steroidal anti-inflammatory drugs and drugs used to teat gout

13. Acetylsalicylic acid tablet, 100-500 mg.
14. Allopurinol tablet, 500 mg
16. Ibuprofen tablet, 200 mg
17. Indomethacin capsule or tablet, 25 mg
18. Paracetamol tablet, 100-500 mg, syrup, 125 mg/5 ml
19. Codeine tablet, 30 mg (phosphate)
20. Morphine inj, 10 mg (sulfate or hydrochloride) in 1-ml ampoule

21. Pethidine inj. 50 mg (hydrochloride) in 1-ml ampoule
22. Buprenorphine tab 200-400 mg inj. 0.3 mg/ml in 1ml ampoule

3. Anntiallergics and drugs used in anaphylaxis

23. Chlorpheniramine tablet, 4 mg (hydrogen maleate) inj. 1mg (hydrogen maleate) in 1-ml ampoule
24. Dexamethasone tablet, 500 ug, 4 mg, Inj. 4 mg (as sodium phosphate) in 1-ml ampoule
25. Epinephrine inj. 1 mg (as hydrochloride) in 1-ml ampoule
26. Hydrocortisone powder for inj. 100 mg (as sodium succinate) in vial
27. Prednisolone tablet, 5 mg.

4. Antidotes and other substances used in poisonings

28. Charcoal, activated powder
29. Desferrioxamine powder for inj. 500 mg (mesilate) in vial
30. Dimercaprol inj. in oil, 50 mg/ml in 2 ml ampoule
31. Naloxone inj., 400 ug (hydrochloride) in 1 ml ampoule
32. Penicillamine Capsule or tablet, 250 mg
33. Sodium calcium edetate inj. 200 mg/ml in 4ml ampoule

5. Antiepileptics

34. Carbamazepine tablet, 100 mg, 200 mg
35. Ethosuximide capsule or tablet, 250 mg syrup, 250 mg / 5 ml
36. Phenobarbital tablet, 30 mg, 60 mg, elixir, 15 mg / 5 ml
37. Phenytoin capsule or tablet, 25 mg, 100 mg (sodium salt) inj. 50 mg (sodium salt) / ml in 5-ml vial
38. Valproic acid enteric coated tablet, 200 mg. 500 mg. (sodium salt)

6. Anti-infective drugs

6.1 Anthelmintics

39. Mebendazole chewable tablet, 100 mg
40. Praziquantel tablet 150 mg, 600 mg
41. Diethylcarbamazine tablet, 50 mg, 100 mg (dihydrogen citrate)

6.2.1 Antibacterials

42. Amoxicillin capsule or tablet, 250 mg, 500 mg (anhydrous)
43. Ampicillin powder for inj., 500 mg (as sodium salt) in vial
44. Benzathine powder for inj. 1.44 g + benzylpenicillin (=2.4 million IU) in 5 ml vial
45. Benzylpenicillin powder for inj. 60 mg (=1 million IU). 3 g (=5 million IU) (as sodium or potassium salt) in vial
46. Cloxacillin capsule, 500 mg (as sodium salt) powder for oral solution, 125 mg (as sodium salt)/5 ml
47. Piperacillin powder for injection, 1 g, 2g (as sodium salt) in vial
48. Procaine powder for injection + benzylpencillin 1 g(= 1million IU), 3 g (= 3 million IU)

6.2.2 Other antibacterials

49. Chloramphenicol capsule, 250 mg; oral suspension, 150 mg (as palmitate salt)/ 5 ml powder for injection.
50. Erythromycin capsule or tablet, 250 mg(as stearate or ethy1 succinate) powder for oral suspension, 125 mg (as stearate or ethy1 succinate) powder for inj. 500 mg (as lactobionate) in vial
51. Gentamicin Inj, 10 mg, 40 mg (as sulfate)/ ml in 2 ml vial
52. Metronidazole tablet, 200-500 mg; inj. 500 mg in 100 ml vial;

oral suspension, 200 mg (as benzoate) / 5 ml

53. Sulfadimidine tablet, 500 mg; oral suspension, 500 mg/ 5 ml; inj. 1 g (sodium salt) in 3 ml ampoule
54. Sulfamethoxazole tablet, 100 mg / 200 mg + trimethoprim 40 mg/ 80 mg; oral suspension 200 mg; 40 mg / 5 ml
55. Tetracycline capsule or tablet, 250 mg (hydrochloride)
56. Ciprofloxacin tablet, 250 mg (as hydrochloride)
57. Doxycycline, capsule or tablet, 100 mg (as hyclate) powder for inj. 100 mg (as hyclate) in ampoule
58. Nitrofurantion tablet, 100 mg
59. Clofazimine capsule, 50 mg, 100 mg
60. Dapsone tablet, 50 mg, 100 mg

6.2.3 Antituberculosis drugs

61. Ethambutol tablet, 100 - 400 mg (hydrochloride)
62. Isoniazid tablet, 100 -300 mg
63. Pyrazinamide tablet, 500 mg
64. Rifampicin capsule or tablet, 150 mg, 300 mg
65. Rifampicin + Isoniazid tablet, 150 mg + 100 mg; 450 mg + 300 mg
66. Streptomycin powder for injection, 1 g (as sulfate) in vial
67. Thioacetazone + isoniazid tablet, 50 mg + 100 mg, 150 mg + 300 mg

6.3 Antifungal drugs

68. Amphotericin - B powder for injection, 50 mg in vial
69. Griseofulvin capsule or tablet, 125 mg, 250 mg
70. Ketoconazole tablet 200 mg; oral suspension, 100 mg / 5 ml

71. Nystatin tablet, 100 000 IU, 500 000 IU

6.4 Antiprotozoal drugs

1. Antiamoebic and antigiardiasis drugs

72. Diloxanitde tablet, 500 mg (furoate)
73. Metronidazole tablet, 200 - 500 mg; inj. 500 mg in 100 ml vial; oral suspension, 200 mg (as benzoate) / 5 ml complementary drug
74. Choloroquine tablet, 150 mg (as phosphate or sulfate)

2. Antileishmaniasis drugs

75. Meglumine antimoniate inj. 30% equivalent to approx, 8.5% antimony, in 5 ml ampoule
76. Pentamidine powder for inj. 200 mg (isetionate) in vial

3. Antimalarial drugs

(a) For curative treatment

77. Primaquine tablet, 7.5 mg , 15 mg (as diphosphate)
78. Quinine tablet, 300 mg (as bisulfate or sulfate); inj. 300 mg (as dihydrochloride) / ml in 2 ml ampoule
79. Sulfadoxine 500 mg + 25 mg pyrimethamine tablet
80. Tetracycline capsule or tablet, 250 mg (hydrochloride)

6.5 Insect repellents

81. Diethyltoluamide topical solution 50%, 75%

7. Antimigraine drugs

82. Ergotamine tablet, 2 mg (tartrate)

8. Antineoplastic and immunosuppressant drugs and drugs used in palliative care

83. Azathioprine tablet, 50 mg; powder for inj. 100 mg (as sodium salt) in vial
84. Cyclosporin capsule, 25 mg; concentrate for inj. 50 mg / ml in 1 ml ampoule
85. Cytotoxic drugs as per WHO list

9. Hormones and antihormones

86. Ethinylestradiol table, 50mg
87. Tamoxifen tablet, 10 mg, 20 mg (as citrate)

10. Antiparkinsonism drugs

88. Levodopa + carbidopa tablet, 100 mg + 10 mg; 250 mg + 25 mg

11. Drugs affecting the blood

89. Ferrous salt tablet, equivalent to 60 mg iron; oral solution, equivalent to 25 mg iron (as sulfate)/ ml
90. Ferrous salt tablet, 60 mg + 250 ug folic acid
91. Folic acid tablet, 1 mg; 5 mg Inj, 1mg (as sodium salt)in 1 ml ampoule
92. Hydroxycobalamin inj. 1 mg in 1 ml ampoule

93. Iron dextran Inj. equivalent to 50 mg iron/ml in 2 ml ampoule
94. Heparin Inj. 1000 IU/ml, 5000 IU/ ml , 20000 IU/ml in 1 ml ampoule
95. Phytomenadione inj, 10 mg/ml in 5 ml ampoule
96. Protamine sulfate inj. 10 mg / ml in 5 ml ampoule
97. Warfarin tablet, 1 mg, 2 mg, 5 mg (sodium salt)

12. Blood products and plasma substitutes

98. Dextran 70 injectable solution, 6%
99. Polygeline injectable solution, 3.5%
100. Albumin, human injectable solution, 5%, 25%
101. Factor VIII concentrate dried
102. Factor IX complex dried (coagulation factors II, VII, IX,X) concentrate

13. Cardiovascular drugs

103. Glyceryl trinitrate tablet (sublingual), 500 ug
104. Isosorbide dinitrate tablet (sublingual), 5 mg
105. Nifedipine capsule or tablet, 10 mg
106. Propranolol tablet, 10 mg, 40 mg (hydrochloride); inj. 1 mg (hydrochloride) in 1 ml ampoule
107. Atenolol Tablet, 50 mg, 100 mg
108. Lidocaine inj. 20 mg (hydrochloride) / ml in 5 ml ampoule
109. Verapamil tablet, 40 mg, 80 mg (hydrochloride); inj. 2.5 mg (hydrochloride) / ml in 2 ml ampoule
110. Procainamide tablet, 250 mg, 500 mg (hydrochloride); inj. 100 mg (hydrochloride)/ ml in 10 ml ampoule
111. Quinidine tablet, 200 mg (sulfate)
112. Hydrochlorothiazide tablet, 25 mg

113. Captopril scored table, 25 mg
114. Methyldopa tablet, 250 mg
115. Resepine tablet, 100 ug, 250 ug
116. Digoxin tablet, 62.5 ug. 250 ug; oral solution 50 ug/ ml; inj. 250 ug/ml in 2ml ampoule
117. Dopamine inj. 40 mg (hydrochloride) / ml in 5 ml vial
118. Streptokinase power for injection, 100 000 IU in vial

14. Dermatological drugs

119. Benzoic acid ointment or cream 6% + 3% salicylic acid
120. Miconazole ointment or cream , 2% (nitate)
121. Nystatin ointment or cream, 100 000 IU/g
122. Sodium thiosulafte solution, 15%
123. Methylrosanilinium aqueous solution 0.5% chloride (gentain violet)
124. Neomycin + bacitracin ointment, 5mg neomycin salfate + 500 IU bacitracin zinc / g
125. Silver sulfadiazine cream, 1% in 500-g container
126. Betamethasone ointment or cream, 0.1% (as valerate)
127. Calamine lotion
128. Hydrocortisone ointment or cream, 1% (acetate)
129. Coal tar solution, topical, 5%
130. Dithranol ointment, 0.1-2%
131. Salicylic acid solution, topical 5%
132. Benzyl benzoate lotion, 25%
133. Permethrin lotion,1%
134. Paraminobenzoic acid cream, lotion or gel-sun protection factor
135. Benzophenones, sun cream, lotion or gel-protection factor
136. Zinc oxide cream or ointment

15. Diagnostic agents

137. Fluorescein eye drops, 1% (sodium salt)
138. Tropicamide eye drops, 0.5%
139. Barium sulfate aqueous suspension
140. Iopanoic acid tablet, 500 mg

16. Disinfectants and antiseptics

141. Chlorhexidine soluiton, 5% (digluconate) for dilution
142. Hydrogen peroxide solution, 1.5%
143. Iodine solution 2.5%
144. Calcium hypochlorite powder (70% available chlorine) for solution

17. Diuretics

145. Furosemide tablet, 40 mg; inj. 10 mg/ ml in 2 ml ampoule
146. Mannitol injectable solution 10%, 20%

18. Gastrointestinal drugs

147. Aluminium hydroxide tablet, 500 mg; oral suspention 320 mg/5 ml
148. Cimetidine tablet, 200 mg
149. Ranitidine tablet 150 mg, 300mg
150. Magnesium hydroxide oral suspension, equivalent to 550 mg magnesium oxide / 10 ml
151. Metoclopramide tablet, 10 mg (as hydrochloride); injection 5 mg / ml in 2 ml ampoule
152. Promethazine tablet, 10 mg, 25 mg (hydrochloride); elixir or syrup, 5 mg (hydrochloride)/5 ml; inj. 25 mg (hydrochloride)/ ml in 2ml ampoule

19. Laxative, anti- inflammatory drug and ORS

153. Sulfasalazine tablet, 500 mg
154. Senna tablet, 7.5 mg (sennosides) (or traditional dosage forms)
155. Oral rehydration salts (for glucose electrolyte solution) powder, 27.9 g/L

Components	g/litre
Sodium chloride	3.5
Trisoldium citrate dihydrate	2.9
Potassium chloride	1.5
Glucose	20.0

20. Hormones, other endocrine drugs and contraceptives

156. Testosterone inj. 200mg (enantate) in1ml ampoule
157. Ethinylestradiol 30 ug/ 50 ug+levonorgestrel 150 ug/ 250 ug tablet
158. Ethinylestradiol 50 ug + 1.0 mg Norethisterone tablet
159. Depot medroxyprogesterone acetate Inj. 150 mg/ml in 1ml and 3ml vials
160. Norethisterone tablet, 350 ug; norethisterone enantate oily solution, 200 mg/ml in 1ml ampoule
161. Copper-containing device
162. Condoms with or without spermicide (nonoxinol)
163. Diaphragms with spermicide (nonoxinol)
164. Ethinylestradiol tablet, 50 μg
165. Insulin inj. (soluble) 40 IU/ml in 10-ml vial, 80 IU/ml in 10ml vial, 100 IU/ml in 10-ml vial
166. Intermediate-acting insulin inj. 40 IU/ml in 10-ml vial. 80- IU/ml in 10-ml vial, 100 IU/ml in 10 ml vial (as compound insulin zinc suspension or, isophane insulin)
167. Tolbutamide Tablet, 500 mg

168. Clomifene tablet, 50 mg (citrate)
169. Norethisterone tablet, 5 mg
170. Levothyroxine tablet, 50 ug, 100 ug (sodium salt)
171. Potassium Iodide tablet, 60 mg
172. Propylthiouracil tablet, 50 mg

21. Immunologicals

173. Tuberculin purified protein derivative (PPD) injection
174. Anti-D immunoglobulin human inj. 250 ug in single-dose vial
175. Antiscorpion sera inj.
176. Antitetanus immunoglobulin human inj. 250 ug in single - dose vial
177. Antivenom sera inj.
178. Diphtheria antitoxin inj. 10000 IU, 20000 IU in vial
179. Immunoglobulin, human normal inj.
180. Rabies Immunoglobulin inj. 150 IU/ml in vial
181. BCG Vaccine (dried) inj.
182. Diphtheria-pertussis- injection tetanus vaccine
183. Diphtheria-tetanus injection vaccine
184. Measles-mumps-rubella injection vaccine
185. Measles vaccine injection
186. Poliomyelitis vaccine injection (inactivated)
187. Poliomyelitis vaccine (live attenuated) oral solution
188. Tetanus vaccine injection
189. Hepatits B vaccine injection
190. Rabies vaccine injection

22. Muscle relazants (peripherally acting) and cholinesterase inhibitors

191. Neostigmine tablet, 15 mg (bromide)

23. Ophthalmological preparations

192. Ciprofloxacin solution eye drops 0.3%
193. Fluorescein - (eye drops) 2% (sodium)
194. Gentamycin solution eyedrops, 2% (sodium)
195. Phyenylephrine solution eye drops, 5%, 10%
196. Pilocarpine - solution eye drops 2%, 4% (hydrochloride or nitrate)
197. Sulphacetamide solution (eye drops), 10%, 20%,30%
198. Timolol solution (eye drops), 0.25%, 0.5% (maleate)

24. Oxytocics

199. Ergometrine tablet, 200 ug (hydrogen maleate) inj. 200 ug (hydrogen maleate) in 1-ml ampoule
200. Oxytocin inj. 10 IU in 1 ml ampoule

25. Psychotherapeutic drugs

201. Amitriptyline tablet, 25 mg (hydrochloride)
202. Chlorpromazine tablet, 100 mg (hydrochloride) syrup, 25 mg (hydrochloride) / 5 ml, inj. 25 mg (hydrochloride)/ ml in 2 ml ampoule
203. Fluphenazine inj. 25 mg (decanoate or enantate) in 1 ml ampoule
204. Haloperidol tablet, 2 mg , 5 mg
205. Lithium carbonate capsule or tablet, 300 mg

26. Drugs acting on the respiratory tract

206. Aminophylline tablet, 100 mg, 200 mg; inj. 25 mg/ml in 10 ml ampoule
207. Beclomethasone inhalation (aerosol), 50 ug (dipropionate) per dose
208. Epinephrine inj. 1 mg (as hydrochloride) in 1 ml ampoule
209. Salbutamol tablet, 2 mg; 4 mg (as sulfate); Inhalation (aerosol), 100 ug (as sulfate) per dose; syrup, 2 mg (as sulfate) / 5 ml; Inj. 50 ug (as sulfate) / ml in 5 ml ampoule; respirator solution for use in nebulizers, 5 mg (as sulfate) / ml
210. Cromoglicic acid inhalation (aerosol), 20 mg (sodium salt) per dose
211. Ephedrine tablet 30 mg (hydrochloride); elixir, 15 mg (hydrochloride)/ 5 ml; inj. 50 mg (sulfate) in 1 ml ampoule
212. Codeine tablet, 10 mg (phosphate)

27. Solutions correcting water, electrolyte and acid-base disturbances

213. Potassium chloride powder for oral solutin
214. Glucose injectable solution, 5% isotonic, 50% hypertonic
215. Glucose with sodium chloride injectable solution, 4% glucose, 0.18% sodium chloride (equivalent to Na^+ 30 mmol/1, Cl^- 30 mmol/1)
216. Potassium chloride 11.2% solution-in 20 ml ampoule (equivalent to K^+ 1.5 mmol/ml, Cl^- 1.5 mmol/ml)
217. Sodium chloride injectable solution, 0.9% isotonic (equivalent to Na^+ 154 mmol/I)
218. Sodium bicarbonate injectable solution, 1.4% isotonic (equivalent to Na^+ 154 mmol/1, HCO_3^- 167 mmol/1) 8.4% solution in 10 ml ampoule (equivalent to Na^+ 1mol/1, HCO_3^- 1 mmol/1)
219. Compound Solution of sodium lactate injectable solution

Prescription Writing and Notes

RATIONAL USE OF DRUGS

Definition :

Rational use of Drugs is the process of providing Essential/Scientific drugs to those people who need them most, in right time, in right dose and at right cost.

India has nearly 6000 pharmaceutical houses producing more than 65000 formulations. About Rs.7000/- crores of drugs are consumed every year. It is acknowledged that substantial proportion of these drugs are irrational combinations which are also wrongly used. Unfortunately the choice of these drugs is influenced significantly by marketing practices of drug companies as has been shown by various studies all over the world. Increased consumption of irrational drugs to maintain the health of industry is counter health. This wastage of scarce resources on hazardous and irrational drugs is something our nation and its people can not afford.

The Rational Drugs must :

1. Meet Real Medical Need

   This means that their use is likely to improve the quality or extent of medical care.

2. Have significant therapeutic value

   This means that drugs must do what is claimed for them, and that patients will benefit from that

3. Be Acceptably Safe

   This means that their likely benefits must out-weigh risks

4. Offer satisfactory value for money

This favours the introduction and use of drugs which work as well as other medicines but cost less.

AREAS WHERE CARE IS NEEDED WHILE PRESCRIBING

Patient based factors :

- Geriatric and paediatric age groups must be prescribed drugs with respect and caution. Adjustment/modification of dosage schedule is at times crucial.
- Pregnant and lactating women must be administered life saving drugs, but little else.
- Should always consider buying capacity of patient.

Medical Factors :

- Avoid polypharmacy as far as possible.
- Consider indications, contraindications, drug interactions and Adverse Drug Reactions.
- Available nonpharmacological modalities of therapy eg. physical exercise, dietary modifications, behavioural therapy and yogic exercises and meditation should be considered before resorting to drug therapy, particularly for diseases like hypertension, diabetes etc.
- Promotional pressures - The subtle ways in which our choice of drug can be influenced is perhaps all-too-well known. This may be tackled in a way that does not deviate from scientific ethics, by mentally formulating a rational prescription in generic terms and then according to preference to the trade name of choice.

Fixed dose combinations :

These contain many unnecessary elements, dose of individual agents may be adequate and dose fixation is almost impossible. Addition of many unnecessary ingredients like vitamins, haematinics etc. may exhorbitantly increase the cost.

The need of the hour is

1. Essential drug list should be made available to prescribers.
2. Identify and weed out irrational combinations from the market.
3. Formulate guidelines for scientific use of specific group of drugs like antibiotics, antihypertensives, analgesics etc.
4. Enforce a uniform regulation for promotional literature.
5. Establishment of Adverse Drug Reaction (ADR) monitoring centre.

Exercise

Students shall critically analyse the drugs prescribed and discuss rationality.

Prescription Writing and Notes

CLINICAL PHARMACOLOGY EXPERIMENTS

The term clincial Pharmacology refers in the broadest sense to any pharmacological activity that is carried out in human beings with the primary objective of making drug therapy better and safer.

Data obtained from animal experiments can not be translated into human therapeutics. The large variation of human population in genetic, enviornmental, nutritional and other background conditions introduce an unfavourable heterogenicity compared to stringent requirements of homogenicity of laboratory animal colonies. Furhter, the impact of illness, both physical and psychological of varying degree, on the pharmacodynamic and pharmcokinetic processes in man compared to high standards of animal health under laboratory conditions complicate the interpretation of many experimental results in clinical pharmacology. Clinical Pharmacology is investigative science. Its objective is to add to the knowledge about human - drug interactions to make drug therapy better and safer.

Human Experimentation has to be undertaken with certain constraints. Thus one cannot have a large sample and for ethical reasons adequate controls also may not be possible. It is essential to have a very high level of quality control in human experimentation. The basic requirements are :

1. Quality of human subject
2. Quality of human treatment and test procedures
3. Quality of evalution of the results.

Some simple test can be performed in clinical Pharmacology by students in the practical classe.

Cold Pressor Test

1. Healthy human volunteers are selected
2. Volunteer will recieve a standard dinner on night before the test and will be housed comfortably.

3. A written informed consent will be obtained and volunteer shifted to the test laboratory maintained at constant temperature.
4. Volunteer will lie down or sit in a reclining chair. Blood pressure and pulse rate will be measured at regular intervals (preferably every 3 minutes by automatic recording device)
5. After the basal stabilization the subjects will immerse one hand in water at 4°C for one minute and effects on blood pressure and pulse rate will be noted for next 15 minutes.
6. Subject will then receive the coded medicine
7. Test will be repeated at 30 min and 60 min.
8. The observer will write his/her impression about the following:
   a) Nature of the drug.
   b) Ettects of the drug.

Observer will discuss findings with teacher incharge.

Effect of drugs on human psychomotor performance

Many drugs are capable of influencing behaviour and psychomotor performance. Human behaviour is so complex that one test can not detect the changes induced by the drug. Therefore a battery of tests is employed for the purpose . This includes the following :

1. **Psychomotor test**
   a) Choice reaction task
   b) Reaction time
   c) Critical flicker fusion
   d) Bimanual co-ordination

2) Mental Function tests

a) Short terms memory-digit span

b) Arithmatic ability

c) Digit-symbol substitution test

3) Subjective Assessment

a) 100 mm visual analogue scale.

Effect of Drugs on human psychomotor performance

Objective : To assess the effect of therapeutic doses of diazepam and caffeine on psychomotor performance.

Subjects : Three healthy volunteers from the class will form one study group. A group of 10-15 students will act as observer.

Students may be divided in as many groups depending upon the number in the class

Study group will be given training

Test : One test each depending upon the facilities in the department may be selected from psychomotor tests and mental function test.

Treatment : Each volunteer will receive one of the following treatments after a control test.

1) Diazepam 2 mg.
2) Caffeine Powder 100 mg.
3) Placebo - glucose powder

Prescription Writing and Notes

DRUG INTERACTIONS

Many Drug Interactions are harmless and many of those which are potentially harmful only occur in a small proportion of patients. Moreover, the severity of interaction show individual variation.Patients at increased risk from drug interactions include those on drugs with small therapeutic ratio, associated renal or hepatic impairment or in elderly age group.

Drug interactions can occur when two or more drugs are given together or can act in the body at the same time. The combination is termed :

HOMERGIC when all the components are active and HETERGIC when only one of the drug is producing response and other is inactive.

Clinically the interactions can also be termed as useful e.g. Sulphamethoxazole + Trimethoprim, unwanted e.g. Tetracycline +Ferrous sulphate, harmful or Adverse Reaction e.g. Warferin + Phenylbutazone.

Sites of Drug Interactions :

Pharmaceutical Interactions :

Taking two interacting drugs together :

- Thiopentone sodium and suxamethonium get precipitated in same syringe.
- Simultaneous addition of heparin and tetracycline in same transfusion bottle leads to complex formation and even precipitation with considerable loss of activity.
- Soluble and protamine zinc insulin (PZI) in same syringe. PZI usually contains excess of protamine which combines with soluble insulin thereby defeating the very purpose of its use.

Pharmacodynamics Interaction :

Occur between drugs with similar or antagonistic pharmacological efffects.They may be due to competition at receptor site or occur between drugs acting on same physiological system. They are predictable from the knowledge of the pharmacology of interacting drugs.

Pharmacokinetic Interactions :

These occur when one drug changes the pharmacological effect of another compound e.g. modifies its onset, intensity or duration of action. This results from alteration in the absorption, distribution, metabolism or excretion thereby increasing or decreasing the amount of drug available for pharmacological effects.

Clinically important drug metabolic interactions

Drug whose metabolism is changed	Interacting drugs	Mechanism of interaction	Clinical consequence	Measures to be taken
Coumarin anticoagulants	Barbiturates Griseofulvin Glutethimide Rifampicin	Enhanced rate of metabolism of coumarin analogues	Decreased anticoagulants effect within a week or so	Combination necessary More frequent check of coagulation. Increase dose of anticoagulant and decrease it after stopping treatment with inducing drug.
Dicoumarol	Clofibrate Chloramphenicol Chlorpropamide Phenyramidol Phenylbutazone	Decreased metabolism of dicoumarol See below	Increased anticoagulants effect (may) occur within a few days	Prophylactic reduction of dicoumarol dose. More frequent check of coagulation. Phenyramidol and chloramphenicol are seldom indicated.
Phenytoin (DPH)	Chloramphenicol Dicoumarol Disulfiram Isoniazid (in slow acetylators) Phenylramidol	Decreased metabolism of phenytoin. Phenytoin and dicoumarol both have concentration dependent kinetics. A small inhibition of their metabolism may result in disproportionate increase in their plasma levels	If plasma level of DPH is too low, the interaction may bring the patient to a more appropriate cocentration. If plasma levels are already optimal, toxicity may result unless DPH-dose is reduced	Keep patient within his appropriate plasma concentration interval, which is usually 10 to 20 mg/ml, but varies with the frequency of seizures. Check plasma concentrations regularly, beginning a week after starting combination therapy.
Tolbutamide	Chloramphenicol Phenylbutazone Phenyramidol	Inhibition of the metabolism of oral antidiabetic drugs	Usually increased hypoglycaemic effect	More frequent checks of blood glucose, and appropriate adjustment of the dose of the antidiabetics.
Chlorpropamide	Chloramphenicol Dicoumarol			

(Contd.)

Drug whose metabolism is changed	Interacting drugs	Mechanism of interaction	Clinical consequence	Measures to be taken
Azathioprine Mercaptopurine	Allopurinol	Allopurinol inhibits xanthine oxidase and hence the metabolism of 6-mercaptopurine (metabolite of azathioprine)	Enhanced effect of the immunosuppresants Toxic effects may occur.	Reduce dose of immuno-suppressants to half or less.
Monoamine oxidase inhibitors	Tyramine (amphetamine)	Increased intraneuronal stores of noradrenaline. Metabolism of oral tyramine blocked.	Tyramine and amphetamine may release high concentrations of noradrenaline and cause dangerous hypertensive reaction and central excitation (amphetamine)	Avoid combination. Dietary instructions.
Doxycycline	Carbamazepine	Enhanced metabolism	Plasma concentration of doxycycline may decrease below minimum inhibitory concentration values	Check that plasma concentrations of doxcycline are appropriate May need more frequent dosing than usually.
Propranolol	Cimetidine	Reduced metabolism	Increased plasma conc.	
	Rifampicin	Increased metabolism	Reduced plasma conc.	
ACE inhibitors	Indomethacin NSAIDS potassium salts	Reduced metabolism	Increased plasma conc.	
	Potassium sparing Diuretics	Increased metabolism	Reduced plasma conc.	
Calcium channel Blockers	Cimetidine	Enzyme induction	Increased plasma conc.	

(Contd.)

Drug whose metabolism is changed	Interacting drug	Mechanism of interaction	Clinical consequences
Verapamil	β Blockers	depressant effect on heart is increased	Asystole, hypotension heart failure
	Rifampicin	Enzyme induction	Reduced plasma concentration
Digoxin	NSAID	Reduced excretion of digoxin	May exacerbate heart failure, reduce GFR & increase plasma digoxin concentration
Aminoglycoside	Ethacrynic Acid, Frusemide, Vancomycin	Increased concentration of Aminoglycosides	Increased ototoxicity
Cephalosporins	Ethacrynic acid, Frusemide, Gentamycin, Vancomycin	Accentuate urinary concent-ration of cephalosporin	Increased nephrotoxicity
Chloramphenicol	Phenobarbitone, Rifampicin	Enzyme induction & metabolism	Reduced plasma concentrations
Heparin	Aspirin, Dipyridamole	Enhancement of anticoagulant effect	Potentiation
Tetracyclines	Antacids	Chelation	Reduced absorption
Lignocaine	Cimetidine	Inhibition of microsomal & enzymes induced metabolism of lignocaine	Increased plasma concentation Risk of toxicity potentiation.

EMERGENCY TREATMENT OF POISONING

All patients who show features of poisoning should be admitted to hospital. Patients who had consumed poisons with delayed action should also be admitted even if they appear well. Delayed action poisons include aspirin, iron, paracetamol, tricyclic antidepressants, diphenoxylate with atropine (Lomotil), and sustained release capsules or tablets.

Only a few poisons such as opioids, paracetamol and iron have specific antidotes and few patients require active removal of poison. Most patients must be treated symptomatically. Knowledge of type of poison helps in anticipating the course of events.

Removal from stomach :

Gastric lavage or emesis is of doubtful value in most cases more than 4 hr after ingestion. Exceptions include aspirin (24 hr), tricyclic antidepressants (8 hr). Chief danger associated with lavage is inhalation of gastric contents and this should not be attempted in drowsy or comatose patients unless cough reflex is present. Airway can be protected by cuffed endotracheal tube.

Emesis can be induced by the ipecacuanha emetic mixture paediatric (BP).

Ipecacuanha liquid extract	0.7	ml
Hydrochloric acid	0.025	ml
Glycerol	1	ml
Syrup	10	ml

Dose : Adult 30 ml, child -18 months 10 ml., other children 15 ml.

Adsorbants :

Given orally, activated charcoal can bind many poisons in stomach, thereby reducing their absorption, but it is effective only if given within 1-2 hr. of ingestion.

Activated Charcoal :

It is safe and is particularly useful for the prevention of absorption of poisons which are toxic in small amounts e.g. antidepressants. The usual adult dose is 50 g every 4 hours.

Active Elimination Techniques :

Techniques intended to enhance the elimination are applicable to a limited number of poisons.

a) Forced alkaline diuresis for salicylates and phenobarbitone.

b) Haemodialysis for salicylates, phenobarbitone, methyl alcohol, ethylene glycol and lithium.
c) Charcoal haemoperfusion for medium and short acting barbiturates, chloral hydrate and meprobamate.

Specific Drugs :

Alcohol :

Features - Ataxia, dysarthria, nystagmus and drowsiness which may progress to coma, with hypotension and acidosis.

Treatment - Maintenance of clear airway
- If hypoglycemia - I.V. glucose

Aspirin :

Features - Hyperventilation, tinnitus, deafness, vasodilatation and sweating, acid-base disturbances and rarely coma.

Treatment - Gastric emptying
- Forced alkaline diuresis

Nonsteroidal antiinflammatory drugs :

Mefenamic acid :

Feature - Convulsions

Treatment - Diazepam

Paracetamol :

Features - Nausea and vomiting, right subcostal pain and tenderness - usually indicates development of hepatic necrosis, liver damage maximal 3-4 days after ingestion and may lead to encephalopathy, haemorrhage, hypoglycemia, cerebral oedema and death.

Treatment - Gastric emptying
- Aetylcysteine
initially 150 mg/kg in 200 ml of 5% glucose over 15 mts.
followed by 50 mg/kg in 500 ml over 4 hr.
then 100 mg/kg in 1000 ml over 16 hr.
- Methionine
2.5 g orally followed by further three doses of 2.5 g every 4 hr.

Narcotic analgesics :

Opioids :

Features - Varying degrees of coma, respiratory depression and pin point pupil.

Coproxamol (combination of dextropropoxyphene and paracetamol)

Features - Those of acute opioid overdosage.
Paracetamol hepatotoxicity may develop later and should be anticipated and treated as indicated above.

Treatment - Naloxone - By continuous intravenous infusion:2 mg diluted in 500 ml.
Infusion rate to adjusted according to the response.
Child - 10 μg/kg; subsequent dose of 100 μg/kg if no response.

Antidepressants

Features - Dry mouth, coma of varying degree, hypotension, hypothermia, hyperreflexia, extensor plantar responses, convulsions, respiratory failure, cardiac conduction defects and arrhythmias. Dilated pupil and urinary retention also occur. Metabolic acidosis may complicate severe poisoning; delirium with confusion, agitation and visual and auditory hallucinations, is common during recovery.

Treatment - Activated charcoal orally.
- I.V. diazepam - May be given orally but large doses required.
- Antiarrhythmic drugs are best avoided.

Hypnotics and anxiolytics :

Barbiturates :

Features - Drowsiness, coma, respiratory depression, hypotension and hypothermia.

Treatment - Forced alkaline diuresis
Charcoal haemoperfusion

Benzodiazepines :

Features - Drowsiness, ataxia, dysarthria and occasionally minor and short lived depression of conciousness.

Treatment - General measures.

Theophylline :

Features - Vomiting (may be severe and intractable), agitation, restlessness, dilated pupils and sinus tachycardia. More serious effects are haematemesis, convulsions and supraventricular and ventricular arrhythmias. Profound hypokalaemia may develop rapidly.

Treatment - Gastric emptying
- Repeated doses of activated charcoal orally.

- I.V. .infusion of potassium chloride for hypokalaemia. E.C.G. monitoring if high doses required.
- I.V. diazepam for convulsions.
- Chlorpromazine/diazepam for sedation in agitated patients.
- In nonasthmatic patients extreme tacycardia, hypokalaemia and hypoglycemia may be reveresed by I.V. administration of propranolol.

Amphetamines :

Features - Wakefulness, excessive activity, paranoia, hallucinations and hypertension followed by exhaustion, convulsions, hypothermia and coma.

Treatment - Chlorpromazine
- If necessary - β-adrenergic blocking agents
  - Tepid sponging
  - I.V. diazepam for convulsions
  - Artificial respiration
  - Forced diuresis

Cyanide poisoning :

Treatment - Dicobalt edetate - 300 mg (20 ml) IV injection over a minute, followed by 50 ml of glucose intravenous infusion 50%, both repeated once or twice if necessary.
- Sodium nitrite 3% (30 mg/ml). 10 ml by IV injection over 3 minutes followed by 25 ml of sodium thiosulphate 50% (50 mg/ml) by I.V. injection over 10 minutes.

Heavy Metals -Poisoning by antimony, arsenic, bismuth gold, mercury, thallium.

Treatment - British Antilewisr it-(BAL) : by intramuscular injection 2.5-3 mg/kg every 4 hr for 2 days.
- 2-4 times on 3rd day.
- 1-2 times daily for 10 days or until recovery.

Poisoning by copper and lead :

Treatment - Penicillamine - 1-2 g daily in divided doses before food until urinary lead is stabilised at less than 500 μg/day; child : 20 mg/kg daily.

Poisoning by lead :

Treatment - Disodium Calcium Edetate - Upto 40 mg/kg twice daily in I.V. saline

(0.9%) infusion for upto 5 days.

Organophosphorus Insecticides (Malathion, TEPP, Parathion dichlorvos, fenthion)

Features - Anxiety, restlessness, dizziness, headache, miosis, nausea, hypersalivation, vomiting, abdominal colic, diarrhoea, bradycardia and sweating are common. Muscle weakness and fasciculations may develop and progress to generalised flaccid paralysis including the ocular and respiratory muscles. Convulsions, coma, pumonary oedema with copius bronchial secretions, hypoxia and arrhythmia occur in severe cases. Hyperglycaemia and glycosuria without ketonuria may also be present.

Treatment - Prevent further exposure by emptying the stomach
- fresh air, clear air way
- removal of bronchial secretions
- adequate ventilation and oxygenation
- removing soiled clothing and washing of contaminated skin.

Atropine sulphate 2 mg IM or IV (according to the severity of poisoning) every 20-30 minutes until skin becomes flushed and dry,pupils dilate and tachycardia develops. Pralidoxime mesylate (PAM) cholinesterase reactivator used as adjunct to atropine, effective only if given within 24 hr.

Pralidoxime mesylate (PAM) - I.M. 1 gm initially followed by 1-2 further doses if necessary.

Slow intravenous injection - 1 gm diluted to 10-15 ml with water given over 5-10 minutes. 1-2 further doses if necessary.

Initial dose may be doubled in very severe poisoning and usual maximum dose is 12 g in 24 hrs.

Folic acid antagonist

Overdosage of methotrexate and folic acid antagonists - calcium leucovorin (3 mg/ml injection). Upto 120 mg IM divided doses over 12 to 24 hr by I.M. or I.V. route. Followed by 15 mg by mouth every 6 hr.

Prescription Writing and Notes

DOSES OF SELECTED EMERGENCY DRUGS

Drug	*Indication*	*Dose*
Adrenaline 1 in 1000 (1 mg/ml)	Anaphylaxis	5 microgram/kg intramuscularly, approximates to : large adult (>100 kg) : 0.75 mL average adults (50-100 kg) : 0.50 mL small adults (<50 kg) : 0.25 mL children : dilute the ampoule in 9 mL of water for injection to give a 1 in 10 000 solution. Inject 0.25 mL per year of age Repeat doses intravenously after 5 minutes if no response.
Aminophylline (250 mg/10 mL)	Asthma not responding to nebulised salbutamol in patients not taking theophylline	adults : 5 mg/kg by slow intravenous injection (over 15-30 minutes)
Atropine (600 microgram/mL)	Symptomatic bradycardia	adult : 300-600 micrograms intravenously
Benztropine (2 mg/2 mL)	Acute dystonia	adult : 1-2 mg intravenously or intramuscularly
Benzylpenicillin (600 mg vial)	Suspected meningococcal infection	Dissolve in water for injections adults : 1.2 g intravenously children under 1 year : 300 mg children 1-9 years : 600 mg intravenously or intramuscularly.
Diazepam (10 mg/2 mL)	Severely distrubed patients Status epilepticus	adults : 5-10 mg by slow intravenous injection adults : 5-10 mg by slow intravenous injection children 1 month-5 years : 0.2-0.5 mg orally 2-5 minutes up to 5 mg children 5 years and older : 1 mg by slow intravenous injection every 2-5 minutes up to 10 mg
Dihydroergotamine (1 mg/mL)	Severe migraine	adults : 1 mg subcutaneously or intramuscularly
Ergometrine (250 microgram/mL)	Bleeding due to incomplete abortion	250 micrograms intramuscularly
Frusemide (20 mg/ 2mL)	Left ventricular failure	20-80 by slow intravenous injection
Glucagon (1 mg)		Dissolve in 1 mL of solvent. Inject subcutaneously, intramuscrlarly or intravenously. adult and children over 25 kg : 1 mg children under 25 kg : 0.5 mg

Drug	*Indication*	*Dose*
Glyceryl trinitrate (400 microgram/spray)	Acute angina	400 microgram sprayed under the tongue. May be repeated once if no response after 5 minutes.
Haloperidol (5 mg/mL)	Acutely disturbed patients	adults : 5-10 mg intramuscularly
Hydrocortisone (100 mg,250 mg)		Dissolve in 2 mL of solvent and inject intravenously over 30 seconds
	Anaphylaxis	2-6 mg/kg depending on the severity of the reaction and after giving adrenaline
	Severe asthma	adults : 200 mg intravenously children : 4 mg/kg intravenously
Lignocaine (100 mg/5 mL)	Sustained ventricular tachycardia	adults : 1 mg/kg intravenously over 1-2 minutes. If successful, begin an infusion at 2-4 mg/minute
Metoclopramide (10 mg/2 mL)	Nausea and vomiting	adults : 10 mg intravenously over 1-2 minutes or intramuscularly
Morphine (15 mg/mL, 30 mg/mL)	Severe pain not due to muscle spasm	adults : 5-20 mg intramuscularly or 5-10 mg by slow intravenous injection children : 0.1-0.2 mg/kg subcutaneously or intramuscularly
Naloxon (2 mg/5 mL)	Narcotic overdose	adults : 0.4-2 mg intravenously. May be repeated after 2-3 minutes children : 0.01 mg/kg intravenously. If no response give 0.1 mg/kg
Pethidine (100 mg/2 mL)	Severe pain	adults : 25-100 mg intramuscularly or 25-50 mg by slow intravenous injection children : 0.5-2 mg/kg intramuscularly
Prochlorperazine (12.5 mg/mL)	Nausea and vomiting, particlarly if due to vestibular disturbances	adults : 12.5 mg intramuscularly
Promethazine (50 mg/2 mL)	Allergic reactions	adults : 25-50 mg intramuscularly (0.5-1 mg/kg can be given intravenously as an adjunctive treatment in anaphylaxis)
Salbutamol for nebulisation (2.5 mg/2.5 mL) (5 mg/2.5 mL)	Acute asthma	adults : 5 mg by nebuliser children 4-12 years : 2.5 mg by nebuliser
Verapamil (5 mg/2 mL)	Paroxysmal supraventricular tachycardia in patients who are not taking beta blockers, are not having an infarction and do not have second or third degree atrioventricular block	adults : 5 mg by slow intravenous injection (1 mg (0.4 mL) per minute). Repeat dose after 5-10 minutes if no response.